MEDITARANEAN
TYPE 2 DIABETES
COOKBOOK
For Seniors

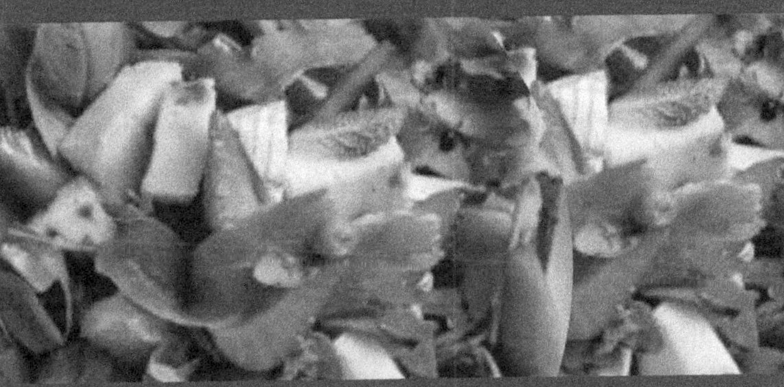

The Ultimate Easy Tasty Low Carb Recipes To Manage And Reverse Type 1 And Type 2 Diabetes

LEONA BUTLER

TABLE OF CONTENT

40 Nutritious Recipes For Mediterranean Type 2 Diabetes Cookbook For Seniors

1. BAKED MEDITERRANEAN CHICKEN WITH ARTICHOKES AND LEMON

2. SEA BASS WITH TOMATO AND OLIVE TAPENADE

3. SPAGHETTI SQUASH WITH TOMATO AND BASIL SAUCE

4. PISTACHIO-CRUSTED SALMON WITH ROASTED VEGETABLES

5. EGGPLANT INVOLTINI WITH RICOTTA AND TOMATO SAUCE

6. QUINOA AND VEGETABLE STUFFED BELL PEPPERS

7. LEMON-OREGANO GRILLED LAMB CHOPS WITH GREEK SALAD

8. GREEK-STYLE TURKEY AND SPINACH MEATBALLS WITH TZATZIKI

9. MEDITERRANEAN ZOODLE BOWL WITH GRILLED CHICKEN

10. SHRIMP AND VEGETABLE SKEWERS WITH HERB MARINADE

Snacks:

1. HUMMUS AND VEGGIE STICKS HUMMUS:

2. GREEK YOGURT WITH HONEY AND WALNUTS

3. ROASTED CHICKPEAS WITH MEDITERRANEAN SPICES

4. CAPRESE SKEWERS WITH CHERRY TOMATOES, MOZZARELLA, AND BASIL

5. OLIVE AND HERB QUINOA CRACKERS

6. BAKED SWEET POTATO FRIES WITH ZA'ATAR

7. ALMOND AND APRICOT ENERGY BITES

8. FETA AND OLIVE TAPENADE ON WHOLE GRAIN CRACKERS

9. GREEK CUCUMBER CUPS WITH TZATZIKI

10. ROASTED RED PEPPER AND WHITE BEAN DIP WITH PITA WEDGES

14-Day Meal Plan

Bonus: 28 Weeks Meal Planner Included

THE PAPERBACK OF THE VERSION HAS A FREE 28 WEEKLY MEAL PLANNER

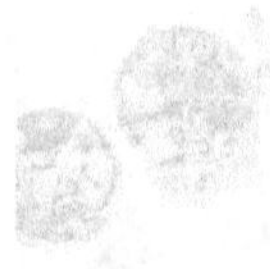

Introduction

Discover a culinary journey to combat type 2 diabetes in seniors with our Mediterranean-inspired cookbook. Tailored for the unique nutritional needs of older adults, this cookbook presents a delectable array of recipes rooted in the renowned Mediterranean diet.

From vibrant salads bursting with nutrient-rich vegetables to hearty mains featuring lean proteins and whole grains, each dish is meticulously crafted to promote blood sugar management and overall well-being.

Embrace the flavors of olive oil, fresh herbs, and lean proteins, seamlessly integrated to create meals that are both health-conscious and irresistibly delicious.

With a focus on simplicity and accessibility, our cookbook empowers seniors to embark on a flavorful and healthful lifestyle, demonstrating that managing diabetes can be a delightful culinary adventure. Elevate your kitchen repertoire and prioritize health without compromising on taste with our Mediterranean Type 2 Diabetes Cookbook for Seniors.

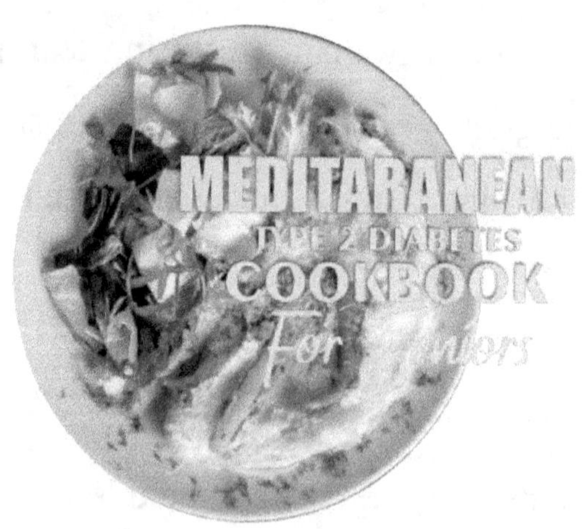

Breakfast

1. Greek Yogurt Parfait with Berries and Nuts

Ingredients:

- cup Greek yogurt
- 1/2 cup mixed berries (blueberries, strawberries, raspberries)
- tablespoons chopped nuts (almonds, walnuts)
- 1 tablespoon honey

Preparation:

1. In a glass or bowl, layer 1/4 cup Greek yogurt.
2. Add a layer of mixed berries.
3. Sprinkle 1 tablespoon of chopped nuts.
4. Drizzle with 1/2 tablespoon honey.
5. Repeat layers.
6. Finish with a drizzle of honey on top.

Nutritional Value:

- Protein: 15g

- Fiber: 5g

- Calories: 250

Cooking Time: Ready in 5 minutes.

2. Mediterranean Omelette with Spinach, Feta, and Tomatoes

Ingredients:

- 4 large eggs

- 1 cup fresh spinach, chopped

- 1/2 cup feta cheese, crumbled

- 1/2 cup cherry tomatoes, halved

- Salt and pepper to taste Olive oil for cooking

Preparation:

1. In a mixing dish, whisk together the eggs and season with salt and pepper.

2. In a skillet over medium heat, heat the olive oil.

3. Add spinach, cook until wilted.

4. Pour eggs over spinach, let set for a minute.

5. Sprinkle feta and tomatoes over the eggs.

6. Gently fold the omelette in half.

7. Cook until eggs are set but still moist inside.

Nutritional Value:

- Calories: Approximately 400

- Protein: 25g

- Fat: 30g

- Carbohydrates: 8g

- Fiber: 2g Cooking Time:

- 10 minutes

3. Whole Grain Toast with Avocado and Smoked Salmon

Ingredients:

- 2 slices of whole grain bread

- ripe avocado

- 100g smoked salmon

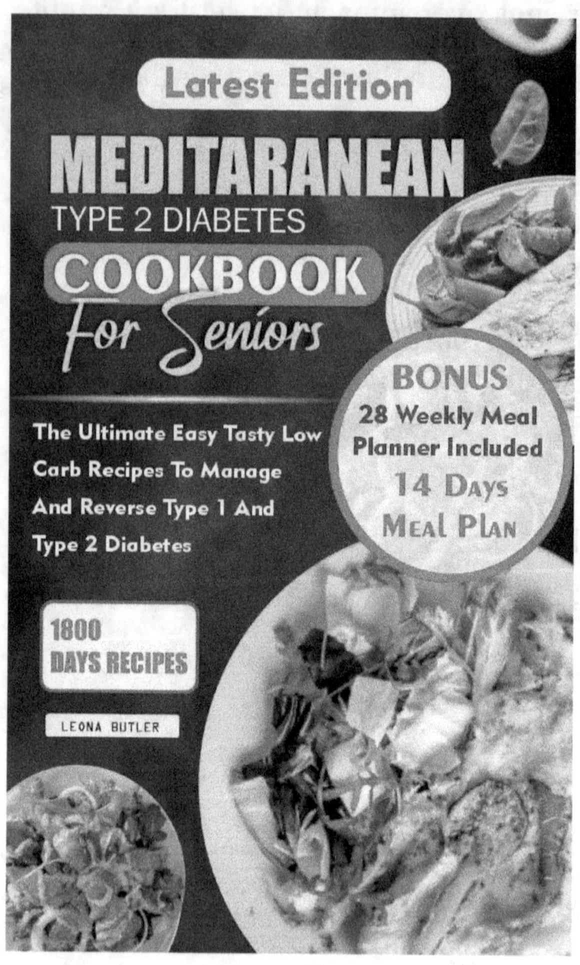

Preparation:

1. Toast the slices of whole grain bread till golden brown.
2. Spread the mashed avocado equally on the toasted bread.
3. Place the smoked salmon on top of the avocado-covered toast. Quantity/Measurement:
4. slices of whole grain bread
5. 1 ripe avocado
6. 100g smoked salmon

Nutritional Value:

- Fiber, vitamins, and minerals are all found in whole grain bread.
- Avocado offers healthy fats, potassium, and vitamins.
- Smoked salmon is rich in protein, omega-3 fatty acids, and B vitamins.

Cooking Time: 5 minutes

4. Quinoa Breakfast Bowl with Roasted Vegetables

Ingredients:

- cup quinoa
- cups mixed vegetables (e.g., bell peppers, cherry tomatoes, zucchini)
- 2 tablespoons olive oil
- Salt and pepper to taste
- 1 teaspoon dried thyme
- 1 teaspoon paprika
- 4 large eggs
- avocado, sliced Fresh parsley for garnish

Preparation:

1. Rinse quinoa thoroughly. Cook with 2 cups water until fluffy.

2. Preheat oven to 400°F (200°C). Toss vegetables with olive oil, salt, pepper, thyme, and paprika.

3. Roast for 20-25 mins.

4. Poach or fry eggs to desired doneness.

5. Assemble bowls: quinoa, roasted veggies, eggs, avocado. Garnish with parsley.

Nutritional Value (per serving):

Calories 480, Protein 16g, Fiber 12g, Healthy Fats 25g. Cooking time: 30 minutes. Enjoy your nutritious quinoa breakfast bowl!

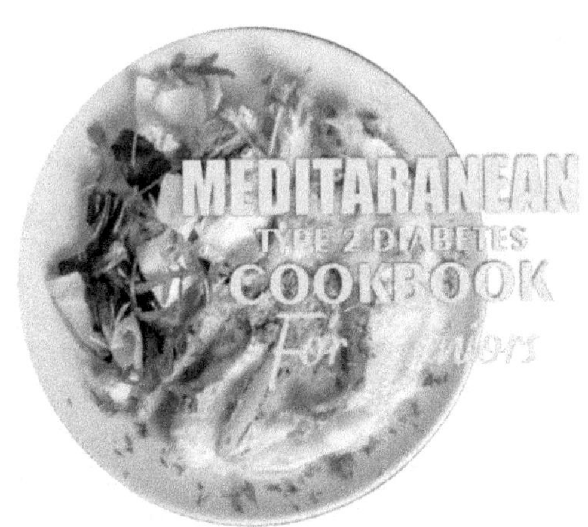

5. Shakshuka with Poached Eggs

Ingredients:

- tbsp olive oil

- onion, diced

- bell peppers, chopped

- garlic cloves, minced

- 1 tsp cumin

- 1 tsp paprika

- 1/2 tsp chili powder

- 1 can (400g) crushed tomatoes

- Salt and pepper to taste

- 4-6 eggs

- Fresh parsley for garnish

Preparation:

1. Heat olive oil in a skillet. Add diced onion, sauté until golden.

2. Add chopped bell peppers and minced garlic, cook until softened.

3. Stir in cumin, paprika, and chili powder. Pour in crushed tomatoes, season with salt and pepper.

4. Simmer for 10-15 minutes.

5. Create small wells in the sauce, crack eggs into them. Cover and poach eggs for 5-7 minutes.

6. Garnish with fresh parsley. Serve hot.

Nutritional Value:

- Calories: Approximately 250 per serving
- Protein: 12g
- Fat: 18g
- Carbohydrates: 15g
- Fiber: 4g Cooking Time:
- Approximately 25-30 minutes

6. Bulgur Porridge with Almonds and Dried Apricots

Ingredients:

- cup bulgur
- cups water
- 1/2 cup chopped almonds
- 1/2 cup dried apricots, diced
- 2 cups milk
- 2 tablespoons honey
- 1/2 teaspoon vanilla extract
- Pinch of salt

Preparation:

1. Rinse bulgur and place it in a pot with water. Bring to a boil, then reduce to a low heat for 10 minutes.

2. Stir in almonds, apricots, milk, honey, vanilla, and salt.

3. Simmer uncovered for an additional 10-15 minutes, or until the bulgur is tender.

4. Adjust consistency with more milk if needed.

5. Serve warm, garnished with additional almonds and apricots.

Nutritional Value:

- Calories: Approximately 350 per serving

- Protein: 10g

- Fiber: 8g

- Healthy fats from almonds

- Rich in vitamins A and C from dried apricots

Cooking Time:

Approximately 20-25 minutes.

7. Mediterranean Egg Muffins with Olives and Sundried Tomatoes

Ingredients:

- 12 large eggs
- 1/2 cup diced black olives
- 1/2 cup chopped sundried tomatoes
- 1/4 cup feta cheese
- 1/4 cup chopped fresh parsley
- 1/2 teaspoon salt
- 1/4 teaspoon black pepper.

Preparation:

1. Preheat oven to 375°F (190°C).
2. In a bowl, whisk eggs and season with salt and pepper.
3. Add olives, sundried tomatoes, feta, and parsley. Mix well.
4. Grease a muffin tin and pour egg mixture evenly into 12 cups.

5. Bake for 20-25 minutes until eggs are set.

6. Allow muffins to cool for 5 minutes before serving.

Nutritional Value (per serving):

- Calories: 120, Protein: 10g, Fat: 8g, Carbohydrates: 2g.

Cooking Time: 20-25 minutes.

8. Sardine and Tomato Bruschetta on Whole Grain Bread

Ingredients:

- can (4.375 oz) of sardines in olive oil
- cups cherry tomatoes, halved
- 2 cloves garlic, minced
- 1/4 cup fresh basil, chopped
- 1 tablespoon extra virgin olive oil
- Salt and pepper to taste 4 slices whole grain bread

Preparation:

1. Drain and flake the sardines, discarding bones.
2. In a bowl, combine sardines, cherry tomatoes, garlic, and basil.
3. Mix in the olive oil, salt, and pepper.
4. Toast whole grain bread slices.
5. Spoon sardine-tomato mixture onto each slice.
6. Drizzle with additional olive oil if desired.

Nutritional Value (per serving):

- Calories: ~300
- Protein: ~15g
- Fat: ~15g
- Carbohydrates: ~30g
- Fiber: ~6g

Cooking Time:

Prep: 15 minutes

Cooking: 5 minutes

9. Lentil and Vegetable Frittata

Ingredients:

- 100g dry green lentils

- 5 large eggs

- cup cherry tomatoes, halved

- 1/2 cup red bell pepper, diced

- 1/2 cup zucchini, diced

- 1/4 cup red onion, finely chopped

- cloves garlic, minced

- 1/2 cup feta cheese, crumbled

- 2 tbsp olive oil

- 1 tsp dried oregano

- Salt and pepper to taste

Nutritional Value:

- Per serving (approximate):

- Calories: 320
- Protein: 20g
- Fat: 18g
- Carbohydrates: 22g
- Fiber: 7g

Preparation:

1. Lentils should be cooked according to package directions, then drained.
2. Preheat oven to 375°F (190°C).
3. In a bowl, whisk eggs and add oregano, salt, and pepper.
4. Heat olive oil in an oven-safe skillet, sauté garlic, onion, bell pepper, and zucchini.
5. Add cooked lentils and tomatoes, stir well.
6. Pour egg mixture over vegetables, sprinkle feta, and let it cook on the stove for 3 minutes.

7. Transfer skillet to the oven, bake for 15-20 minutes or until eggs are set. Slice, serve, and enjoy your nutritious Lentil and Vegetable Frittata!

10. Orange and Almond Flour Pancakes

Ingredients:

- cup almond flour
- 1/2 cup orange juice
- large eggs
- 2 tablespoons honey
- 1 teaspoon baking powder
- 1/2 teaspoon vanilla extract
- 1/4 teaspoon salt
- Zest of 1 orange
- Butter or oil for cooking

Nutritional Value:

- Per serving (approximate):
- Calories: 220
- Protein: 8g
- Fat: 16g
- Carbohydrates: 14g
- Fiber: 3g
- Sugars: 8g

Preparation:

1. In a bowl, whisk almond flour, baking powder, and salt.
2. In another bowl, mix orange juice, eggs, honey, vanilla extract, and orange zest.
3. Combine wet and dry ingredients until a batter forms.
4. Heat a pan, add butter or oil.
5. Pour 1/4 cup of batter per pancake onto the pan.

6. Cook until golden brown, about 2-3 minutes per side.

7. Serve warm and enjoy your nutritious orange and almond flour pancakes!

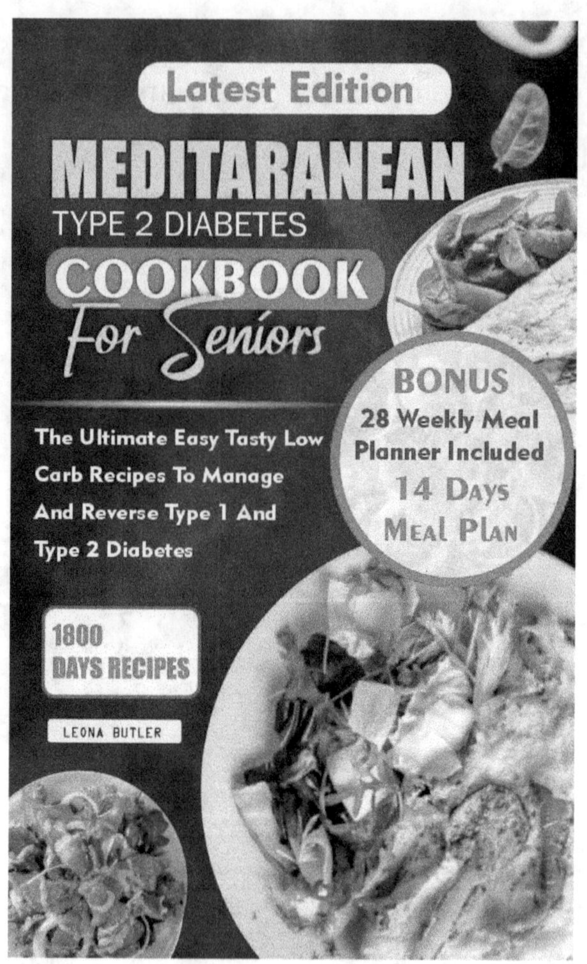

Latest Edition
MEDITARANEAN
TYPE 2 DIABETES
COOKBOOK
For Seniors
The Ultimate Easy Tasty Low
Carb Recipes To Manage
And Reverse Type 1 And
Type 2 Diabetes
BONUS
28 Weekly Meal
Planner Included
14 Days
Meal Plan
1800
DAYS RECIPES
LEONA BUTLER

Lunch:

1. Grilled Chicken Greek Salad with Feta and Kalamata Olives

Ingredients:

- 2 boneless, skinless chicken breasts

- 1 tablespoon olive oil

- Salt and pepper to taste

- 1 teaspoon dried oregano

- 4 cups mixed salad greens

- 1 cup cherry tomatoes, halved

- 1 cucumber, sliced

- 1/2 red onion, thinly sliced

- 1/2 cup crumbled feta cheese 1/4 cup Kalamata olives, pitted

Preparation:

1. Preheat grill to medium-high heat.

2. Rub chicken breasts with olive oil, season with salt, pepper, and oregano.

3. Grill the chicken for 6-8 minutes per side, or until done.

4. Let chicken rest, then slice into strips.

5. In a large bowl, combine salad greens, tomatoes, cucumber, red onion, feta, and olives.

6. Top with grilled chicken strips.

7. Toss salad gently to combine.

Nutritional Value:

- Approximate serving size: 1/4 of the recipe

- Calories: 350

- Protein: 30g

- Fat: 18g

- Carbohydrates: 20g

- Fiber: 5g

- Sugars: 8g Sodium: 700mg

Cooking Time:

Total time: 25 minutes (including grill preheating and chicken resting).

2. Quinoa and Chickpea Stuffed Peppers

Ingredients:

- 4 large bell peppers
- 1 cup quinoa
- 1 can chickpeas (15 oz)
- 1 cup diced tomatoes
- cup diced red onion
- cloves garlic, minced
- 1 teaspoon cumin
- 1 teaspoon paprika
- Salt and pepper to taste
- 1 cup vegetable broth 1 cup shredded cheese (optional)

Preparation:

1. Preheat oven to 375°F (190°C).

2. Cut tops off peppers, remove seeds, and blanch in boiling water for 5 minutes.

3. Cook quinoa according to package instructions.

4. Sauté onions and garlic until translucent. Add chickpeas, tomatoes, cumin, paprika, salt, and pepper.

5. Mix in cooked quinoa and vegetable broth, simmer for 5 minutes.

6. Stuff peppers with the quinoa-chickpea mixture, top with cheese.

7. Bake for 25-30 minutes, or until the peppers are soft. Nutritional Value:

8. Approximate per serving: Calories 350, Protein 14g, Fat 5g, Carbs 65g, Fiber 12g. Cooking Time:

9. 45-50 minutes from start to finish.

3. Mediterranean Tuna Salad with White Beans and Cherry Tomatoes

Ingredients:

- 1 can (6 oz) tuna, drained
- 1 can (15 oz) white beans, rinsed and drained
- cup cherry tomatoes, halved
- 1/4 cup red onion, finely chopped
- tablespoons Kalamata olives, sliced
- tablespoons capers 1/4 cup fresh parsley,

chopped Dressing:

- tablespoons olive oil
- 2 tablespoons red wine vinegar
- 1 teaspoon Dijon mustard Salt and pepper to taste

Preparation:

1. In a large bowl, combine tuna, white beans, cherry tomatoes, red onion, olives, capers, and parsley.
2. In a separate bowl, whisk together olive oil, red wine vinegar, Dijon mustard, salt, and pepper for the dressing.
3. Toss the salad lightly with the dressing to mix.
4. Refrigerate for at least 30 minutes to allow flavors to combine.
5. Serve chilled.

Nutritional Value (per serving):

- Calories: Approximately 350
- Protein: 25g
- Fat: 15g
- Carbohydrates: 30g
- Fiber: 8g

Cooking Time:

Preparation: 15 minutes

Refrigeration: 30 minutes

4. Eggplant and Zucchini Lasagna with Ground Turkey

Ingredients:

- Eggplant and Zucchini Lasagna:

- 2 medium-sized eggplants

- 2 large zucchinis

- pound ground turkey

- cups marinara sauce

- 1 cup ricotta cheese

- cup shredded mozzarella cheese

- 1/2 cup grated Parmesan cheese

- cloves garlic, minced

- 1 teaspoon dried oregano Salt and pepper to taste

Preparation:

1. Preheat oven to 375°F.
2. Slice eggplants and zucchinis thinly, sprinkle with salt, and let sit for 15 minutes.
3. Brown ground turkey with minced garlic, salt, and pepper.
4. Layer eggplant and zucchini slices, ground turkey, marinara sauce, ricotta, and cheeses in a baking dish.
5. Repeat layers, finishing with a cheese layer on top.
6. 30–35 minutes, or until golden and bubbling.

Nutritional Value:

Per serving (approximate): Calories: 350, Protein: 25g, Fat: 20g, Carbohydrates: 18g.

Cooking Time:

Approximately 1 hour.

5. Lemon-Herb Marinated Grilled Shrimp Skewers with Quinoa

Ingredients:

- pound large shrimp, peeled and deveined

- tablespoons olive oil

- 2 tablespoons lemon juice

- 2 cloves garlic, minced

- 1 teaspoon dried oregano

- 1 teaspoon dried thyme

- Salt and pepper to taste Wooden skewers, soaked in water

Preparation:

1. In a bowl, mix olive oil, lemon juice, minced garlic, oregano, thyme, salt, and pepper.

2. Add shrimp to the marinade, coating evenly. Refrigerate for at least 30 minutes.

3. Thread marinated shrimp onto skewers.

4. Preheat grill to medium-high heat.

5. Grill shrimp skewers for 2-3 minutes per side until opaque.

6. Serve over cooked quinoa.

Nutritional Value (per serving):

- Calories: 250

- Protein: 30g

- Fat: 12g

- Carbohydrates: 10g

- Fiber: 2g

Cooking Time: Approximately 10 minutes.

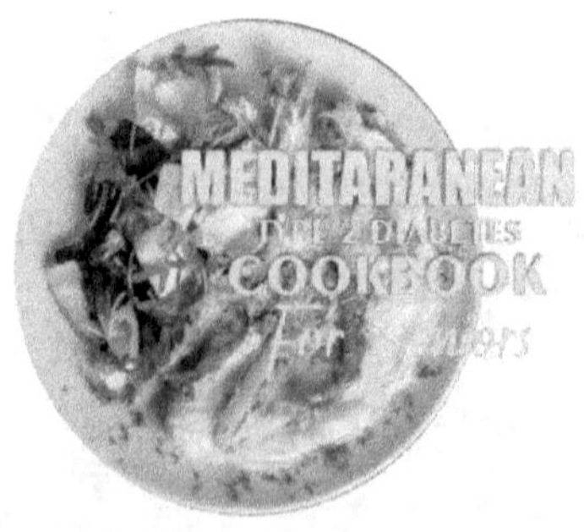

6. Roasted Vegetable and Hummus Wrap

Ingredients:

- cup mixed vegetables (zucchini, bell peppers, cherry tomatoes)
- tbsp olive oil
- Salt and pepper to taste
- 4 whole wheat tortillas
- 1 cup hummus
- Fresh greens (spinach, lettuce)

Preparation:

1. Preheat oven to 400°F (200°C).
2. Toss vegetables with olive oil, salt, and pepper to taste. Roast for 20-25 minutes until tender.
3. Spread hummus on each tortilla.
4. Divide roasted vegetables among tortillas.
5. Top with fresh greens.
6. Roll into wraps.

Nutritional Value (per serving):

- Calories: 350

- Protein: 10g

- Fiber: 8g Healthy

- fats: 15g

Cooking Time: 25 minutes

7. Baked Cod with Mediterranean Salsa

Ingredients:

- 4 cod fillets (about 6 oz each)

- 2 tbsp olive oil

- 1 tsp dried oregano

- Salt and pepper to taste

Mediterranean Salsa:

- cup cherry tomatoes, diced

- 1/2 cup cucumber, diced

- 1/4 cup red onion, finely chopped

- tbsp Kalamata olives, sliced

- 2 tbsp fresh parsley, chopped

- 1 tbsp olive oil

- 1 tbsp red wine vinegar Salt and pepper to taste

Preparation:

1. Preheat oven to 400°F (200°C).

2. Arrange the cod fillets on a baking sheet. Drizzle with olive oil and season with oregano, salt, and pepper to taste. Bake for 15-20 minutes, or until the fish easily flakes.

3. Combine tomatoes, cucumber, red onion, olives, and parsley in a mixing dish. Combine the olive oil, red wine vinegar, salt, and pepper in a mixing bowl. Combine thoroughly.

4. Serve baked cod topped with Mediterranean salsa.

Nutritional Value (per serving):

- Calories: 320
- Protein: 30g
- Fat: 16g
- Carbohydrates: 10g
- Fiber: 2g

Cooking Time: 25 minutes

8. Spinach and Feta Turkey Burger on Whole Wheat Bun

Ingredients:

- Ground turkey (1 lb)
- Spinach (1 cup, chopped)
- Feta cheese (1/2 cup, crumbled)
- Whole wheat buns (4

- Salt (1/2 tsp)

- Black pepper (1/4 tsp)

- Garlic powder (1/2 tsp)

- Olive oil (1 tbsp)

Preparation:

1. In a bowl, combine ground turkey, chopped spinach, crumbled feta, salt, black pepper, and garlic powder.

2. Divide the mixture into 4 portions and shape into burger patties.

3. In a skillet over medium heat, heat the olive oil.

4. Cook turkey patties for 5-6 minutes per side or until fully cooked.

5. Toast whole wheat buns in the skillet for 1-2 minutes.

Nutritional Value (per serving):

Calories: 350, Protein: 30g, Carbohydrates: 25g, Fat: 16g, Fiber: 4g.

Cooking Time:

Approximately 12-15 minutes.

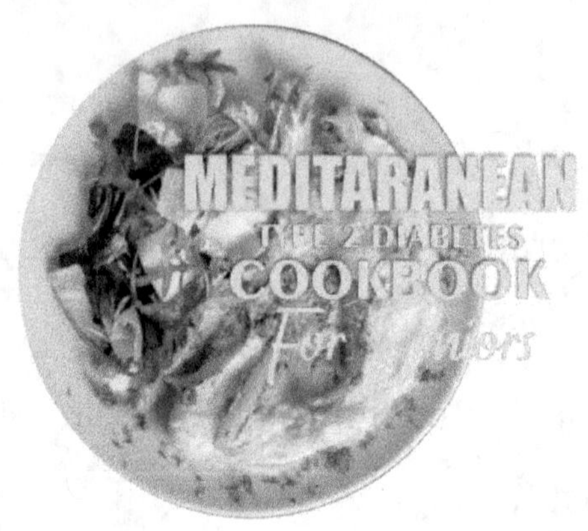

9. Greek Lentil Soup with Spinach and Lemon

Ingredients:

- 1 cup dried green lentils

- onion, finely chopped

- carrots, diced

- celery stalks, chopped

- garlic cloves, minced

- 1 teaspoon dried oregano

- 1 teaspoon ground cumin

- 4 cups vegetable broth

- 4 cups fresh spinach, chopped

- 1 lemon, juiced Salt and pepper to taste

Preparation:

1. Rinse lentils and set aside.

2. Sauté onions, carrots, and celery in a saucepan until softened.

3. Add garlic, oregano, and cumin; cook for 1 minute.

4. Pour in vegetable broth and add lentils. Simmer for 20-25 minutes.

5. Stir in spinach and cook until wilted.

6. Add lemon juice, salt, and pepper.

7. Serve hot, enjoying a nutritious, flavorful Greek Lentil Soup.

Cooking time: 30 minutes.

Nutritional value: Rich in fiber, protein, and vitamins.

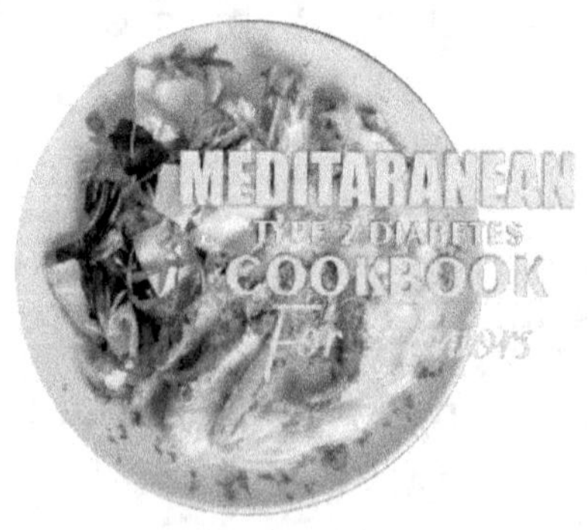

10. Stuffed Grape Leaves with Ground Lamb and Rice

Ingredients:

- 1 cup long-grain rice

- 1/2 pound ground lamb

- 1/4 cup pine nuts

- 1/4 cup chopped fresh mint

- 1/4 cup chopped fresh parsley

- onion, finely chopped

- cloves garlic, minced

- 1/4 cup olive oil

- 1 teaspoon ground allspice

- 1 teaspoon ground cinnamon

- Salt and pepper to taste 1 jar grape leaves, drained

Preparation:

1. Cook rice according to package instructions.

2. In a skillet, sauté lamb, pine nuts, onion, and garlic in olive oil until browned.

3. Mix in cooked rice, mint, parsley, allspice, cinnamon, salt, and pepper.

4. Place grape leaves flat, fill with mixture, and roll tightly.

5. Arrange rolls in a pot, cover with water, and simmer for 30 minutes. Serve and enjoy these nutritious, flavorful stuffed grape leaves!

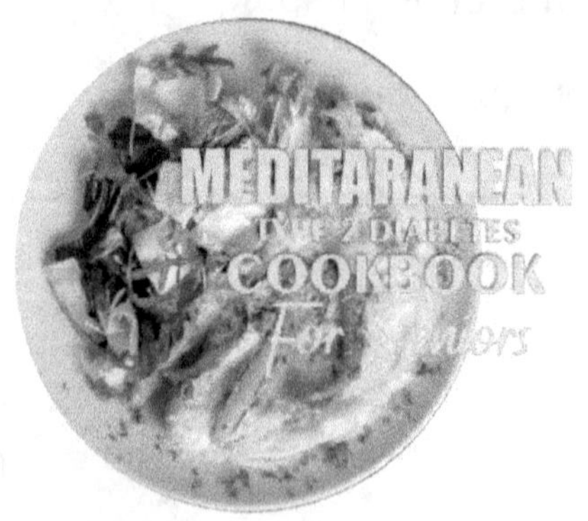

Dinner:

1.Baked Mediterranean Chicken with Artichokes and Lemon

Ingredients:

- 4 boneless, skinless chicken breasts

- 1 can (14 oz) drained and quartered artichoke hearts

- 1 lemon, thinly sliced

- 1/4 cup olive oil

- 4 cloves garlic, minced

- 1 teaspoon dried oregano

- Salt and black pepper to taste

- 1/2 cup cherry tomatoes, halved

- 1/4 cup Kalamata olives, pitted and sliced Fresh parsley for garnish

Nutritional Value:

- High in protein from chicken.
- Good fats from olive oil.
- Rich in fiber and vitamins from artichokes and tomatoes.

Preparation:

1. Preheat oven to 375°F (190°C).
2. Season chicken with salt, pepper, and oregano.
3. In a baking dish, arrange chicken, artichokes, lemon slices, tomatoes, and olives.
4. Whisk together olive oil and minced garlic, then pour over the chicken.
5. Bake for 25-30 minutes, or until the chicken is thoroughly done. Garnish with fresh parsley before serving.

2. Sea Bass with Tomato and Olive Tapenade

Ingredients:

- 4 sea bass fillets (6 oz each)

- 2 cups cherry tomatoes, halved

- 1/2 cup Kalamata olives, pitted and chopped

- 2 tablespoons capers, drained

- 2 cloves garlic, minced

- 1/4 cup fresh parsley, chopped

- 2 tablespoons olive oil Salt and pepper to taste

Preparation:

- Preheat oven to 400°F (200°C).

- In a bowl, mix tomatoes, olives, capers, garlic, parsley, and olive oil.

- Season sea bass with salt and pepper, then place on a baking sheet.

- Top fillets with the tomato and olive mixture.

- Bake for 15-20 minutes or until fish flakes easily. Serve immediately, garnished with extra parsley.

Nutritional Value:

Approximately 300 calories per serving.

Rich in Omega-3 fatty acids and protein.

Cooking Time:

15-20 minutes.

3. Spaghetti Squash with Tomato and Basil Sauce

Ingredients:

- spaghetti squash

- cups tomato sauce

- 1/4 cup fresh basil, chopped

- 2 cloves garlic, minced

- 1 tablespoon olive oil

- Salt and pepper to taste
- Grated Parmesan cheese (optional)

Preparation:

1. Preheat oven to 375°F (190°C).
2. Remove the seeds from the spaghetti squash and cut it in half lengthwise. Drizzle with olive oil and season with salt and pepper.
3. Place squash on a baking sheet, cut side down, and bake for 40-45 minutes.
4. In a pan, sauté garlic in olive oil until fragrant.
5. Add tomato sauce, simmer for 15 minutes.
6. Once squash is done, use a fork to scrape out "spaghetti" strands.
7. Toss squash with tomato sauce, add fresh basil.
8. Serve with Parmesan cheese if desired.

Nutritional Value:

- Approximate serving: 1 cup
- Calories: 120
- Carbohydrates: 20g
- Protein: 2g
- Fat: 4g
- Fiber: 5g

4. Pistachio-Crusted Salmon with Roasted Vegetables

Ingredients:

- Salmon fillets (4, 6 oz each)
- Pistachios (1 cup, finely chopped)
- Olive oil (3 tbsp)
- Lemon juice (2 tbsp)
- Dijon mustard (1 tbsp) Salt and pepper to taste

Preparation:

1. Preheat oven to 400°F (200°C).

2. In a bowl, mix chopped pistachios, olive oil, lemon juice, Dijon mustard, salt, and pepper.

3. Pat salmon dry, spread pistachio mixture on top.

4. Place salmon on a baking sheet, bake for 15-18 minutes.

Roasted Vegetables:

Ingredients:

- Assorted vegetables (carrots, broccoli, bell peppers, 4 cups)
- Olive oil (2 tbsp)
- Garlic powder (1 tsp)
- Italian seasoning (1 tsp) Salt and pepper to taste

Preparation:

1. Toss vegetables with olive oil, garlic powder, Italian seasoning, salt, and pepper.

2. Spread on a separate baking sheet, roast for 20-
    25 minutes.

Nutritional Value:

Salmon: High in omega-3 fatty acids, protein. Each
fillet approx. 350 calories.

Pistachios: Good source of healthy fats, protein,
fiber. 1 cup around 700 calories.

Roasted Vegetables: Low-calorie, rich in vitamins.
Mix provides about 150 calories per serving.

Cooking Time:

Salmon: 15-18 minutes.

Vegetables: 20-25 minutes.

5. Eggplant Involtini with Ricotta and Tomato Sauce

Ingredients:

- 2 large eggplants

- 1 cup ricotta cheese

- 1 cup grated Parmesan cheese

- egg

- cups marinara sauce

- 1 teaspoon olive oil

- Salt and pepper to taste Fresh basil for garnish

Preparation:

1. Preheat oven to 375°F (190°C).

2. Slice eggplants lengthwise into thin strips. Set aside for 15 minutes after sprinkling with salt. Mix ricotta, Parmesan, and egg in a bowl. Spread the mixture on eggplant slices and roll them up.

3. Place rolled eggplants in a baking dish, cover with marinara sauce, and drizzle with olive oil.

4. 25-30 minutes, or until golden and bubbling.

5. Garnish with fresh basil before serving.

Nutritional Value:

- Calories: Approximately 250 per serving

- Protein: 12g

- Fat: 15g

- Carbohydrates: 20g

- Fiber: 5g

Cooking Time:

25-30 minutes

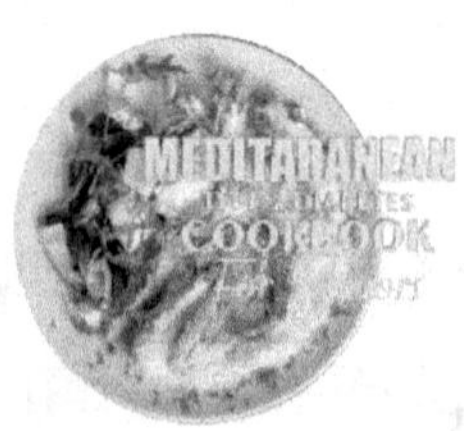

6. Quinoa and Vegetable Stuffed Bell Peppers

Ingredients:

- 4 large bell peppers
- cup quinoa
- cups vegetable broth
- 1 cup black beans, cooked
- 1 cup corn kernels
- cup diced tomatoes
- 1/2 cup diced red onion
- 1/2 cup diced zucchini
- cloves garlic, minced
- 1 teaspoon cumin
- 1 teaspoon paprika
- Salt and pepper to taste 1 cup shredded cheese (optional)

Preparation:

1. Preheat oven to 375°F (190°C).

2. Cut tops off bell peppers, remove seeds, and blanch in boiling water for 5 minutes.

3. Cook quinoa in vegetable broth according to package instructions.

4. In a pan, sauté garlic, onions, and zucchini until softened.

5. Mix cooked quinoa, black beans, corn, tomatoes, cumin, paprika, salt, and pepper in a bowl.

6. Stuff bell peppers with the quinoa mixture.

7. Top with shredded cheese if desired.

8. Bake for 25-30 minutes, or until the peppers are soft.

Nutritional Value:

Approximate per serving:

- Calories: 350

- Protein: 15g

- Fat: 5g

- Carbohydrates: 60g

- Fiber: 10g

- Sugars: 8g

- Sodium: 600mg

Cooking Time:

45-50 minutes (including prep and baking).

7. Lemon-Oregano Grilled Lamb Chops with Greek Salad

Ingredients:

For Lemon-Oregano Grilled Lamb Chops:

- 4 lamb chops

- 2 tbsp olive oil

- 2 tbsp lemon juice

- 2 tsp dried oregano

- Salt and pepper to taste

For Greek Salad:

- 2 cups cherry tomatoes, halved
- 1 cucumber, diced
- 1/2 red onion, thinly sliced
- 1 cup feta cheese, crumbled
- 1/4 cup Kalamata olives
- 3 tbsp olive oil
- 2 tbsp red wine vinegar
- 1 tsp dried oregano Salt and pepper to taste

Preparation:

1. Marinate lamb chops in olive oil, lemon juice, oregano, salt, and pepper for 30 mins.
2. Grill chops for 3-4 mins per side until desired doneness.
3. Combine tomatoes, cucumber, red onion, feta, and olives for the salad.

4. In a separate bowl, whisk together olive oil, red wine vinegar, oregano, salt, and pepper.

5. Toss the salad with the dressing.

Nutritional Value:

Lamb Chops: High in protein, iron, and B vitamins.

Greek Salad: Rich in vitamins, antioxidants, and healthy fats.

Cooking Time:

Lamb Chops: 10 minutes.

Greek Salad: No cooking required.

8. Greek-Style Turkey and Spinach Meatballs with Tzatziki

Ingredients:

- Lean ground turkey - 1 pound

- Fresh spinach, finely chopped - 1 cup

- Red onion, finely diced - 1/2 cup

- Garlic, minced - 2 cloves

- Feta cheese, crumbled - 1/2 cup

- Egg - 1

- Breadcrumbs - 1/2 cup

- Dried oregano - 1 teaspoon

- Salt and pepper - to taste

Preparation:

1. Preheat oven to 375°F (190°C).

2. In a bowl, mix ground turkey, chopped spinach, red onion, garlic, feta, egg, breadcrumbs, oregano, salt, and pepper.

3. Shape the mixture into meatballs and lay them on a baking pan.

4. Bake for 20-25 minutes until golden and cooked through.

Tzatziki Sauce:

Ingredients:

- Greek yogurt - 1 cup

- Cucumber, grated and drained - 1/2 cup
- Garlic, minced - 1 clove
- Fresh dill, chopped - 1 tablespoon
- Lemon juice - 1 tablespoon
- Salt and pepper - to taste

Preparation:

1. Combine Greek yogurt, grated cucumber, minced garlic, chopped dill, lemon juice, salt, and pepper in a bowl.
2. Stir well and chill for at least 30 minutes before serving.

Nutritional Value:

- Per serving (4 meatballs with tzatziki):
- Calories: 300
- Protein: 28g
- Carbohydrates: 15g

- Fat: 15g

- Fiber: 3g

Cooking Time:

Approximately 45 minutes.

9. Mediterranean Zoodle Bowl with Grilled Chicken

Ingredients:

Zoodles:

- 4 medium zucchinis, spiralized

- tablespoon olive oil Salt and pepper to taste

Grilled Chicken:

- boneless, skinless chicken breasts

- 2 tablespoons olive oil

- teaspoon dried oregano Salt and pepper to taste

Mediterranean Sauce:

- 1/4 cup feta cheese, crumbled

- tablespoons lemon juice
- 1 tablespoon fresh parsley, chopped 1 clove garlic, minced

Preparation:

1. Toss zoodles with olive oil, salt, and pepper. Set aside.
2. Mix olive oil, oregano, salt, and pepper. Coat chicken and grill for 15-20 minutes.
3. Combine feta, lemon juice, parsley, and garlic for the sauce.

Nutritional Value:

Approximate per serving: 400 calories, 25g protein, 20g fat, 10g carbs.

Cooking Time:

30 minutes. Enjoy your healthy Mediterranean Zoodle Bowl with Grilled Chicken

10. Shrimp and Vegetable Skewers with Herb Marinade

Ingredients:

- lb large shrimp, peeled and deveined

- cups assorted vegetables (bell peppers, cherry tomatoes, zucchini), chopped

- 1/4 cup olive oil

- 2 tablespoons fresh lemon juice

- 2 cloves garlic, minced

- 1 tablespoon fresh parsley, chopped

- 1 teaspoon fresh thyme leaves Salt and pepper to taste Marinade

Preparation:

1. In a bowl, mix olive oil, lemon juice, minced garlic, chopped parsley, thyme, salt, and pepper.

2. Save some of the marinade for basting while grilling.

3. Thread shrimp and vegetables onto skewers, brushing with the herb marinade.

4. Marinate for 30 minutes.

Cooking:

5. Preheat grill to medium-high heat.

6. Grill skewers for 4-5 minutes per side, basting with reserved marinade.

7. Cook until shrimp are opaque and vegetables are tender.

Nutritional Value (per serving):

- Calories: 280
- Protein: 20g
- Fat: 18g
- Carbohydrates: 12g
- Fiber: 3g

Cooking Time: 20 minutes

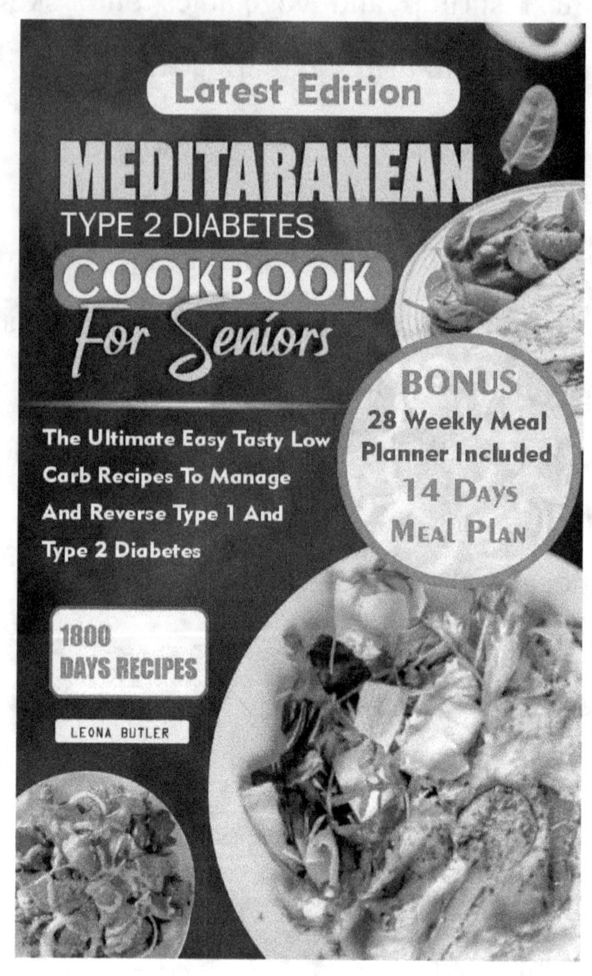

Latest Edition
MEDITARANEAN
TYPE 2 DIABETES
COOKBOOK
For Seniors
The Ultimate Easy Tasty Low Carb Recipes To Manage And Reverse Type 1 And Type 2 Diabetes
BONUS
28 Weekly Meal Planner Included
14 Days Meal Plan
1800 DAYS RECIPES
LEONA BUTLER

Snacks:

1. Hummus and Veggie Sticks
Hummus:

Ingredients:

- 1 can (15 oz) chickpeas (drained)

- 1/4 cup tahini

- 1/4 cup olive oil

- clove garlic

- tablespoons lemon juice

- 1/2 teaspoon cumin

- Salt to taste

- 2-3 tablespoons water (adjust for consistency)

Preparation:

1. Combine all ingredients in a food processor.

2. Blend until smooth.

3. Adjust salt and consistency.

4. Serve drizzled with olive oil.

Nutritional Value (per serving):

- Calories: ~150

- Protein: ~5g

- Fiber: ~4g

- Healthy fats: ~10g

Cooking Time: 10 minutes

Veggie Sticks:

Ingredients:

- Carrot sticks

- Cucumber sticks

- Bell pepper strips Cherry tomatoes

Preparation:

1. Wash and cut veggies into sticks or strips.

2. Arrange on a plate.

Nutritional Value (per serving):

Calories: ~30

Fiber: ~3g

Vitamins and minerals from veggies.

Combine hummus and veggie sticks for a delicious, nutritious snack.

2. Greek Yogurt with Honey and Walnuts

Ingredients:

- cup Greek yogurt
- tablespoons honey 1/4 cup chopped walnuts

Preparation:

1. In a bowl, scoop out 1 cup of Greek yogurt.
2. Drizzle 2 tablespoons of honey over the yogurt.
3. Sprinkle with 1/4 cup chopped walnuts.
4. Gently mix the ingredients to ensure an even distribution.

Nutritional Value:

- Calories: Approximately 300

- Protein: 15g

- Fat: 20g

- Carbohydrates: 20g

- Fiber: 2g

3. Roasted Chickpeas with Mediterranean Spices

Ingredients:

- 2 cans (15 oz each) drained and washed chickpeas

- 2 tablespoons olive oil

- 1 teaspoon ground cumin

- 1 teaspoon smoked paprika

- 1/2 teaspoon garlic powder 1/2 teaspoon onion powder

- 1/2 teaspoon dried oregano Salt and pepper to taste

Preparation:

1. Preheat oven to 400°F (200°C).

2. Pat chickpeas dry with a paper towel.

3. In a bowl, toss chickpeas with olive oil, cumin, paprika, garlic powder, onion powder, oregano, salt, and pepper.

4. Place chickpeas in a single layer on a baking sheet.

5. Roast in the preheated oven for 25-30 minutes, shaking the pan halfway through, until chickpeas are golden and crispy.

6. Allow to cool before serving.

Nutritional Value:

- Serving Size: 1/2 cup
- Calories: 160

- Protein: 6g

- Fiber: 5g

- Fat: 8g

- Carbohydrates: 18g

- Sodium: 240mg

Cooking Time: 25-30 minutes

4. Caprese Skewers with Cherry Tomatoes, Mozzarella, and Basil

Ingredients:

- Cherry Tomatoes (1 pint)

- Fresh Mozzarella Balls (8 oz)

- Fresh Basil Leaves (1 bunch)

- Balsamic Glaze (2 tbsp)

- Olive Oil (2 tbsp) Salt and Pepper to taste

Preparation:

1. Wash cherry tomatoes and basil leaves.

2. Thread one cherry tomato, one mozzarella ball, and one basil leaf onto each skewer.

3. Arrange skewers on a serving platter.

4. Drizzle with olive oil, then drizzle with balsamic glaze and season with salt and pepper.

5. Allow flavors to meld for 15 minutes.

6. Serve and enjoy the refreshing Caprese Skewers.

Nutritional Value:

- Calories: Approximately 120 per serving

- Fat: 9g

- Protein: 7g

- Carbohydrates: 3g

- Fiber: 1g

Cooking Time:

- Preparation: 15 minutes

- Marinating: 15 minutes

5. Olive and Herb Quinoa Crackers

Ingredients:

- 100g quinoa
- cup water
- tbsp olive oil
- 1/2 cup mixed herbs (rosemary, thyme, oregano)
- 1/4 cup black olives, chopped
- 1/2 cup whole wheat flour 1/2 tsp salt

Preparation:

1. Rinse quinoa, then cook in water until tender.
2. Preheat oven to 350°F (175°C).
3. In a bowl, mix cooked quinoa, olive oil, herbs, olives, flour, and salt.
4. Knead into a dough and roll it out thinly.
5. Cut into cracker shapes and place on a baking sheet. Bake for 15-20 minutes, or until the edges are brown.

6. Allow to cool before serving.

Nutritional Value (per serving):

- Calories: 120

- Protein: 4g

- Fat: 6g

- Carbohydrates: 14g

- Fiber: 2g

Cooking Time: 30 minutes (including preparation)

6. Baked Sweet Potato Fries with Za'atar

Ingredients:

- 2 large sweet potatoes, peeled and cut into fries

- 2 tablespoons olive oil

- 1 tablespoon za'atar spice 1 teaspoon salt
  Preparation:

- Preheat the oven to 425°F (220°C).

- In a bowl, toss sweet potato fries with olive oil, za'atar, and salt until evenly coated.

- Place the fries on a baking pan in a single layer.

- Bake for 25-30 minutes, flipping halfway, until golden and crisp.

- Remove from the oven and let them cool for a few minutes before serving.

Nutritional Value:

Calories: Approximately 200 per serving

Fiber: 4g

Vitamin A: 400% DV Healthy fats from olive oil

Cooking Time: 25-30 minutes

7. Almond and Apricot Energy Bites

Ingredients:

- Almond and Apricot Energy Bites

- 1 cup almonds

- cup dried apricots

- 1/2 cup rolled oats

- tablespoons honey

- 1 teaspoon vanilla extract A pinch of salt

Preparation:

1. In a food processor, blend almonds until finely chopped.

2. Add apricots, oats, honey, vanilla extract, and salt.

3. Pulse until the mixture is well combined.

4. Form small balls using the mixture and place them on a tray.

5. Refrigerate for at least 30 minutes.

Nutritional Value:

- Serving Size: 1 Energy Bite

- Calories: Approximately 80

- Protein: 2g

- Carbohydrates: 10g

- Fat: 4g

- Fiber: 2g

Cooking Time:15 minutes

Refrigeration: 30 minutes

8. Feta and Olive Tapenade on Whole Grain Crackers

Ingredients:

- 1 cup crumbled feta cheese

- cup pitted Kalamata olives

- 1/4 cup extra-virgin olive oil

- tablespoons capers

- 2 cloves garlic, minced

- 1 teaspoon lemon zest

- 1 tablespoon lemon juice

- 1/4 teaspoon black pepper Whole grain crackers

Preparation:

1. In a food processor, combine feta, olives, olive oil, capers, garlic, lemon zest, lemon juice, and black pepper.

2. Pulse until a coarse paste forms.

3. Adjust seasoning to taste.

4. Refrigerate for at least 30 minutes.

5. Serve on whole grain crackers.

- Nutritional Value (per serving):

- Calories: 120

- Fat: 10g

- Protein: 3g

- Carbohydrates: 4g

- Fiber: 1g

Cooking Time: 10 minutes (excluding refrigeration)

9. Greek Cucumber Cups with Tzatziki

Ingredients:

- 4 large cucumbers

- cup Greek yogurt

- 1/2 cup diced red onion

- 1/2 cup diced tomatoes

- 1/4 cup chopped fresh dill

- cloves garlic, minced

- 1 tablespoon olive oil

- 1 tablespoon lemon juice Salt and pepper to taste

Preparation:

1. Cucumber Cups: Cut cucumbers into 2-inch sections, hollow out the centers with a spoon to form cups.

2. Tzatziki: In a bowl, combine Greek yogurt, red onion, tomatoes, dill, garlic, olive oil, lemon juice, salt, and pepper. Mix well.

3. Assembly: Fill cucumber cups with tzatziki
    mixture.

4. Serve: Garnish with additional dill. Refrigerate
    for at least 30 minutes.

Nutritional Value:

Each serving provides approximately 120 calories,
8g protein, 7g fat, and 10g carbohydrates.

Cooking Time:

Preparation takes 15 minutes, plus refrigeration
time.

10. Roasted Red Pepper and White Bean Dip with Pita Wedges

Ingredients:

- can (15 oz) washed and drained white beans

- roasted red peppers, peeled and seeded

- 2 cloves garlic, minced

- 2 tablespoons olive oil

- 1 tablespoon lemon juice

83

- 1 teaspoon cumin Salt and pepper to taste

Preparation:

1. In a food processor, combine white beans, roasted red peppers, garlic, olive oil, lemon juice, cumin, salt, and pepper.

2. Blend until smooth, adjusting seasoning to taste.

3. Transfer the dip to a serving bowl.

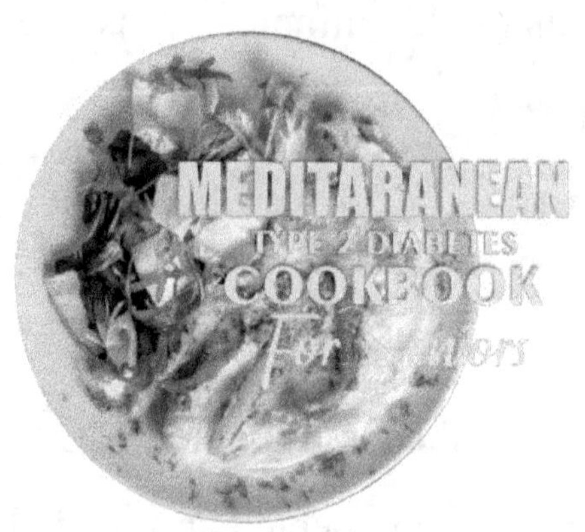

Nutritional Value:

- Serving Size: 2 tablespoons
- Calories: 60
- Protein: 2g
- Fat: 3g
- Carbohydrates: 7g
- Fiber: 2g

Pita Wedges:

- 4 whole wheat pita bread, cut into wedges
- 1 tablespoon olive oil 1/2 teaspoon paprika
- Salt to taste

Preparation:

1. Preheat oven to 400°F (200°C).
2. In a bowl, toss pita wedges with olive oil, paprika, and salt.

3. Spread the wedges on a baking sheet and bake for 8-10 minutes or until golden and crisp.

Nutritional Value:

- Serving Size: 1/4 of the recipe

- Calories: 120

- Protein: 3g

- Fat: 4g

- Carbohydrates: 18g

- Fiber: 3g

Cooking Time:

Dip: 10 minutes

Pita Wedges: 10 minutes

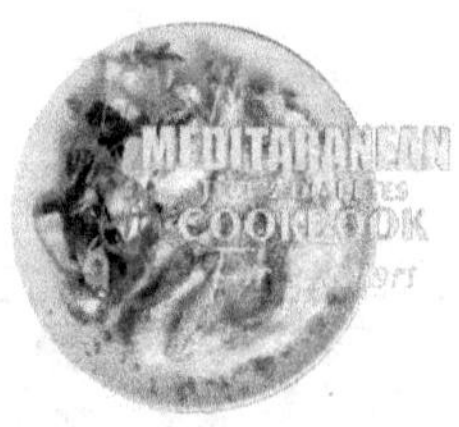

14 - DAY MEAL PLAN

Day 1:

Breakfast: Greek Yogurt Parfait with Berries and Nuts

Lunch: Grilled Chicken Greek Salad with Feta and Kalamata Olives

Dinner: Baked Mediterranean Chicken with Artichokes and Lemon

Snack: Hummus and Veggie Sticks

Day 2:

Breakfast: Mediterranean Omelette with Spinach, Feta, and Tomatoes

Lunch: Quinoa and Chickpea Stuffed Peppers

Dinner: Sea Bass with Tomato and Olive Tapenade

Snack: Greek Yogurt with Honey and Walnuts

Day 3:

Breakfast: Whole Grain Toast with Avocado and Smoked Salmon

Lunch: Mediterranean Tuna Salad with White Beans and Cherry Tomatoes

Dinner: Spaghetti Squash with Tomato and Basil Sauce

Snack: Roasted Chickpeas with Mediterranean Spices

Day 4:

Breakfast: Quinoa Breakfast Bowl with Roasted Vegetables

Lunch: Eggplant and Zucchini Lasagna with Ground Turkey

Dinner: Pistachio-Crusted Salmon with Roasted Vegetables

Snack: Caprese Skewers with Cherry Tomatoes, Mozzarella, and Basil

Day 5:

Breakfast: Shakshuka with Poached Eggs

Lunch: Lemon-Herb Marinated Grilled Shrimp Skewers with Quinoa

Dinner: Eggplant Involtini with Ricotta and Tomato Sauce

Snack: Olive and Herb Quinoa Crackers

Day 6:

Breakfast: Bulgur Porridge with Almonds and Dried Apricots

Lunch: Roasted Vegetable and Hummus Wrap

Dinner: Quinoa and Vegetable Stuffed Bell Peppers

Snack: Baked Sweet Potato Fries with Za'atar

Day 7:

Breakfast: Mediterranean Egg Muffins with Olives and Sundried Tomatoes

Lunch: Baked Cod with Mediterranean Salsa

Dinner: Lemon-Oregano Grilled Lamb Chops with Greek Salad

Snack: Almond and Apricot Energy Bites

Repeat this cycle for Days 8-60, ensuring a variety of meals for each day to maintain a balanced and nutritious diet.

Bonus: 28 Weeks Meal Planner Included

MY WEEKLY MEAL PLANNER

Date

	Breakfast	Lunch	Dinner
MON			
TUE			
WED			
THU			
FRI			
SAT			
SUN			

SHOPPING LIST:

TO DO LIST

NOTES AND TIPS

Conclusion

In conclusion, this Mediterranean Type 2 Diabetes Cookbook for seniors offers a holistic approach to managing diabetes through flavorful and nutritious recipes.

The carefully curated collection emphasizes the health benefits of a Mediterranean diet, rich in fresh fruits, vegetables, whole grains, and heart-healthy fats. These recipes not only cater to the specific dietary needs of seniors with Type 2 diabetes but also embrace the cultural richness and diverse flavors associated with the Mediterranean region.

By incorporating these delicious and balanced meals into their daily routine, seniors can take proactive steps towards better blood sugar control and overall well-being. The thoughtful selection of ingredients ensures that each recipe not only tastes delightful but also supports a diabetic-friendly lifestyle.

As you embark on this culinary journey, remember that adopting and adapting to this Mediterranean-inspired diet is not just a prescription for health but a celebration of life. Empower yourself with the knowledge that every meal is an opportunity to nourish your body and savor the joy of good food. Embrace this lifestyle change not as a restriction, but as a delicious and fulfilling commitment to your health.

Let the vibrant flavors and nutritional benefits inspire you to make this transformative choice, taking charge of your diabetes journey with vitality and deliciousness. Your well-being deserves the richness of a Mediterranean feast – savor it with each mindful bite!

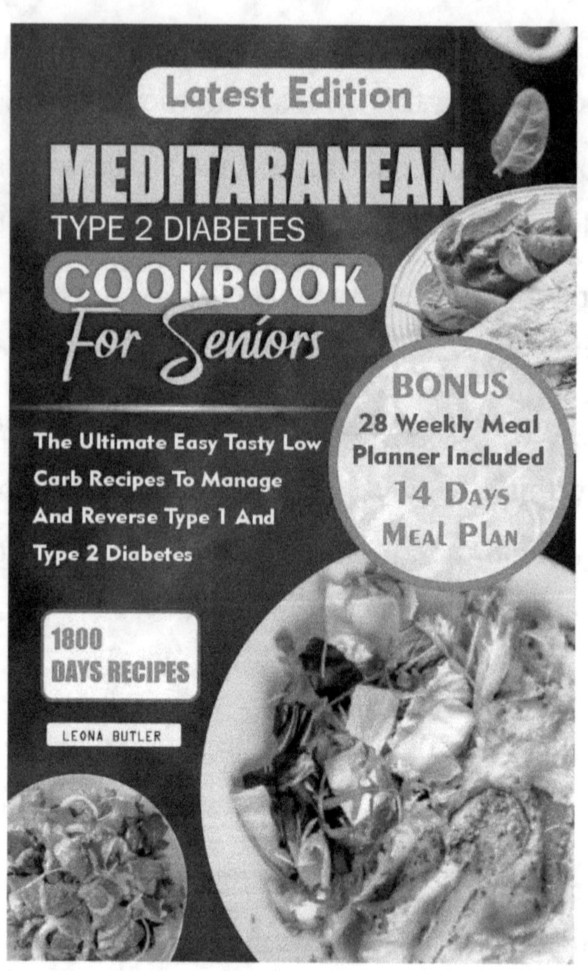

Latest Edition
MEDITARANEAN
TYPE 2 DIABETES
COOKBOOK
For Seniors
The Ultimate Easy Tasty Low Carb Recipes To Manage And Reverse Type 1 And Type 2 Diabetes
BONUS
28 Weekly Meal Planner Included
14 Days Meal Plan
1800 DAYS RECIPES
LEONA BUTLER

MY WEEKLY MEAL PLANNER

Date

	Breakfast	Lunch	Dinner
MON			
TUE			
WED			
THU			
FRI			
SAT			
SUN			

SHOPPING LIST:

- ....
- ....
- ....
- ....

TO DO LIST

....

....

....

....

NOTES
AND TIPS

MY WEEKLY MEAL PLANNER

Date

	Breakfast	Lunch	Dinner
Mon			
Tue			
Wed			
Thu			
Fri			
Sat			
Sun			

SHOPPING LIST:

- ⚫ ··································
- ⚫ ··································
- ⚫ ··································
- ⚫ ··································

To Do List

··································

··································

··································

··········

Notes and Tips

MY WEEKLY MEAL PLANNER

Date

	Breakfast	Lunch	Dinner
MON			
TUE			
WED			
THU			
FRI			
SAT			
SUN			

SHOPPING LIST:

To Do List

- ....
- ....
- ....
- ....

NOTES
AND TIPS

MY WEEKLY MEAL PLANNER

Date

	Breakfast	Lunch	Dinner
MON			
TUE			
WED			
THU			
FRI			
SAT			
SUN			

SHOPPING LIST:

- ·····························
- ·····························
- ·····························
- ·····························

To Do List

·····················

·····················

·····················

···········

NOTES AND TIPS

MY WEEKLY MEAL PLANNER

Date

	Breakfast	Lunch	Dinner
MON			
TUE			
WED			
THU			
FRI			
SAT			
SUN			

SHOPPING LIST:

TO DO LIST

NOTES AND TIPS

MY WEEKLY MEAL PLANNER

Date

	Breakfast	Lunch	Dinner
MON			
TUE			
WED			
THU			
FRI			
SAT			
SUN			

SHOPPING LIST:

TO DO LIST

- ....
- ....
- ....
- ....

NOTES AND TIPS

MY WEEKLY MEAL PLANNER

Date

	Breakfast	Lunch	Dinner
Mon			
Tue			
Wed			
Thu			
Fri			
Sat			
Sun			

SHOPPING LIST:

To Do List

- - - - - - - - - - - - - - - -

Notes And Tips

MY WEEKLY MEAL PLANNER

Date

	Breakfast	Lunch	Dinner
MON			
TUE			
WED			
THU			
FRI			
SAT			
SUN			

SHOPPING LIST:

To Do List

NOTES
AND TIPS

MY WEEKLY MEAL PLANNER

Date

	Breakfast	Lunch	Dinner
Mon			
Tue			
Wed			
Thu			
Fri			
Sat			
Sun			

SHOPPING LIST:

- ....
- ....
- ....
- ....

To Do List

....

....

....

....

Notes And Tips

MY WEEKLY MEAL PLANNER

Date

	Breakfast	Lunch	Dinner
MON			
TUE			
WED			
THU			
FRI			
SAT			
SUN			

SHOPPING LIST:

To Do List

- ....
- ....
- ....
- ....

NOTES
AND TIPS

MY WEEKLY MEAL PLANNER

Date

	Breakfast	Lunch	Dinner
MON			
TUE			
WED			
THU			
FRI			
SAT			
SUN			

SHOPPING LIST:

-
-
-
-

To Do List

NOTES AND TIPS

MY WEEKLY MEAL PLANNER

Date

	Breakfast	Lunch	Dinner
MON			
TUE			
WED			
THU			
FRI			
SAT			
SUN			

SHOPPING LIST:

To Do List

- ● - - - - - - - - - - - - - - - - -   - - - - - - - - - - - - -
- ● - - - - - - - - - - - - - - - - -   - - - - - - - - - - - - -
- ● - - - - - - - - - - - - - - - - -   - - - - - - - - - - - - -
- ● - - - - - - - - - - - - - - - - -   - - - - - - - - - - - -

NOTES
AND TIPS

MY WEEKLY MEAL PLANNER

Date

	Breakfast	Lunch	Dinner
MON			
TUE			
WED			
THU			
FRI			
SAT			
SUN			

SHOPPING LIST:

To Do List

-
-
-
-

NOTES AND TIPS

MY WEEKLY MEAL PLANNER

Date

	Breakfast	Lunch	Dinner
MON			
TUE			
WED			
THU			
FRI			
SAT			
SUN			

SHOPPING LIST:

To Do List

NOTES AND TIPS

MY WEEKLY MEAL PLANNER

Date

	Breakfast	Lunch	Dinner
MON			
TUE			
WED			
THU			
FRI			
SAT			
SUN			

SHOPPING LIST:

To Do List

NOTES AND TIPS

MY WEEKLY MEAL PLANNER

Date

	Breakfast	Lunch	Dinner
MON			
TUE			
WED			
THU			
FRI			
SAT			
SUN			

SHOPPING LIST:

- ....
- ....
- ....
- ....

To Do List

....
....
....
....

NOTES
AND TIPS

MY WEEKLY MEAL PLANNER

Date

	Breakfast	Lunch	Dinner
MON			
TUE			
WED			
THU			
FRI			
SAT			
SUN			

SHOPPING LIST:

TO DO LIST

-
-
-
-

NOTES AND TIPS

MY WEEKLY MEAL PLANNER

Date

	Breakfast	Lunch	Dinner
MON			
TUE			
WED			
THU			
FRI			
SAT			
SUN			

SHOPPING LIST:

TO DO LIST

NOTES
AND TIPS

MY WEEKLY MEAL PLANNER

Date

	Breakfast	Lunch	Dinner
MON			
TUE			
WED			
THU			
FRI			
SAT			
SUN			

SHOPPING LIST:

-
-
-
-

TO DO LIST

NOTES AND TIPS

MY WEEKLY MEAL PLANNER

Date

	Breakfast	Lunch	Dinner
MON			
TUE			
WED			
THU			
FRI			
SAT			
SUN			

SHOPPING LIST:

-
-
-
-

To Do List

NOTES AND TIPS

MY WEEKLY MEAL PLANNER

Date

	Breakfast	Lunch	Dinner
MON			
TUE			
WED			
THU			
FRI			
SAT			
SUN			

SHOPPING LIST:

- ....
- ....
- ....
- ....

TO DO LIST

....

....

....

....

NOTES AND TIPS

MY WEEKLY MEAL PLANNER

Date

	Breakfast	Lunch	Dinner
MON			
TUE			
WED			
THU			
FRI			
SAT			
SUN			

SHOPPING LIST:

-
-
-
-

TO DO LIST

NOTES AND TIPS

MY WEEKLY MEAL PLANNER

Date

	Breakfast	Lunch	Dinner
Mon			
Tue			
Wed			
Thu			
Fri			
Sat			
Sun			

SHOPPING LIST:

- ....
- ....
- ....
- ....

To Do List

....
....
....
....

Notes And Tips

MY WEEKLY MEAL PLANNER

Date

	Breakfast	Lunch	Dinner
MON			
TUE			
WED			
THU			
FRI			
SAT			
SUN			

SHOPPING LIST:

To Do List

- • ....
- • ....
- • ....
- • ....

NOTES
AND TIPS

MY WEEKLY MEAL PLANNER

Date

	Breakfast	Lunch	Dinner
MON			
TUE			
WED			
THU			
FRI			
SAT			
SUN			

SHOPPING LIST:

To Do List

-
-
-
-

NOTES AND TIPS

MY WEEKLY MEAL PLANNER

Date

	Breakfast	Lunch	Dinner
MON			
TUE			
WED			
THU			
FRI			
SAT			
SUN			

SHOPPING LIST:

To Do List

- ....
- ....
- ....
- ....

NOTES
AND TIPS

MY WEEKLY MEAL PLANNER

Date

	Breakfast	Lunch	Dinner
MON			
TUE			
WED			
THU			
FRI			
SAT			
SUN			

SHOPPING LIST:

TO DO LIST

-      - - - - - - - - - - - - - - - -

-      - - - - - - - - - - - - - - - -

-      - - - - - - - - - - - - - - - -

-      - - - - - - - - - - - -

NOTES AND TIPS

MY WEEKLY MEAL PLANNER

Date

	Breakfast	Lunch	Dinner
MON			
TUE			
WED			
THU			
FRI			
SAT			
SUN			

SHOPPING LIST:

TO DO LIST

- • - - - - - - - - - - - - - - - - - - -
- • - - - - - - - - - - - - - - - - - - -
- • - - - - - - - - - - - - - - - - - - -
- • - - - - - - - - - - - - - - - - - - -

NOTES AND TIPS